THE KITCHEN FOR BRAIN HEALTH

NOURISHING RECIPES AND

LIFESTYLE HABITS TO

SAFEGUARD AGAINST

ALZHEIMER'S

Dr. Harmony Wells

INTRODUCTION

Brain Health Essentials

Welcome to the realm of Brain Health Essentials, where we investigate how the decisions we make on a daily basis can maintain and improve our mental health. Consider it a helpful manual for nurturing your brain to become a happier, healthier version of yourself. We'll talk about the importance of brain health in this introduction, particularly in relation to averting conditions like Alzheimer's disease. We're keeping things light and airy, so don't worry! Let's begin with the fundamentals. "You are what you eat" is a proverb that many have heard. It's kind of accurate, though, in terms of your brain! We are going to discuss the amazing nutrients that your brain needs to function properly. It's similar to treating your brain like a tiny VIP. Now picture your brain as a superhero, and consider the nutrients we discuss as its dependable henchmen. We will learn about these nutritional superheroes, including their vitamins, minerals, antioxidants, and omega-3 fatty acids. Warning: They are all here to assist you in becoming the protagonist of your own mental narrative. But there's still more! We'll explore the tasty realm of meals that improve cognitive function. Consider fatty fish as seafaring buddies equipped with the beneficial effects of omega-3 fatty acids, and berries as little antioxidant superheroes. And who can overlook our green friends, the greatest protectors of nutrients—our leafy greens? Then, we'll add some flavor (pun intended) with herbs like turmeric and sage and rosemary, which are known to improve memory. Who knew, after all, that your kitchen could be an undiscovered weapon in the fight for a sound mind? However, it goes beyond just what's in your plate. We'll venture into the realm of Mindful Living and learn how regular movement and stress reduction are like giving your brain a daily high five. Let's get down to business now. Our culinary creations are not only delicious but also beneficial to your brain. It's simple to eat for brain health; all you need to do is enjoy delicious cuisine that will nourish your brain as well. We'll conclude with some useful advice, discuss general wellbeing, and serve as your go-to resource for any difficult queries you may have. So fasten your seatbelt! Our goal is to maximize the happiness of your brain through a straightforward and amiable experience. A happy brain is a healthy brain, so get ready to embrace Brain Health Essentials!

CHAPTER ONE

Nutrient-Rich Foods

Key Ingredients

Welcome to the gastronomic realm of brain health, where we will be delving deeply into the dietary treasures that can strengthen your mental faculties and promote cognitive wellness. Consider this your helpful, all-inclusive guide to designing a kitchen that stimulates the mind!

1. The Nutrients Avengers:

- Minerals and vitamins: The hidden heroes of brain health are these. Think of vitamin B as your brain's performance coach, encouraging it to reach its maximum potential. Important minerals that are necessary for nerve transmission and general cognitive function include iron, zinc, and magnesium.

- **Antioxidants:** Your brain's super heroes in the battle against oxidative stress and inflammation. They maintain the resilience and freshness of your neural environment; they are the cleanup team. Antioxidant-rich berries are like the special guests at this brain party.

-Omega-3 Fatty Acids: Your brain's cells communicate with each other effortlessly thanks to these communication specialists. Omega-3 fatty acids, found in fatty fish like salmon and trout, are the ocean's soldiers that protect cell membrane integrity and promote overall brain function.

2. Highlighted Components on Your Plate:

-Berries: In addition to being delicious, blueberries, strawberries, and raspberries are a great source of antioxidants that help shield your brain from inflammation and oxidative stress. They resemble the colorful artists taking center stage at your all-time favorite concert.

- **Fatty Fish:** Omega-3 fatty acids, especially DHA and EPA, which are vital for brain function, are abundant in salmon, mackerel, and trout. These fats maintain the integrity of brain tissue and facilitate effective neuronal communication. Think of them as the main course on the menu in your brain.

- **Leafy Greens:** Rich in vitamins, minerals, and antioxidants, spinach, kale, and broccoli are the nutritional powerhouses. They are the adaptable performers who take on different parts to assist different brain physiological processes.

3. Herbs and Spices: The Tasty Allies

-Turmeric: Meet the hippest person on the street. Curcumin, the main ingredient in turmeric, possesses strong antioxidant and anti-inflammatory qualities. Not only does it give your food color, but it also adds a plethora of health advantages.

- Rosemary and sage: These herbs are noted for their ability to improve memory in addition to their flavor. Including them in your food improves taste and strengthens brain function. Consider them to be the knowledgeable elders directing your mind toward improved memory.

4. Allies in Lifestyle:

- Exercise: Consider your regular physical activity to be a mental workout. It improves blood flow, encourages the development of new neurons, and supports brain health in general. Your brain enjoys joining this upbeat dancing party.

- Stress Management: Prolonged stress might impede your brain's function. Your brain may relax and rejuvenate itself using techniques like deep breathing, meditation, or even picking up soothing hobby. This self-care regimen is something your brain deserves.

In summation, putting together this all-star cast of nutritional superheroes is necessary to create a kitchen that supports brain health. You're not just feeding your body when you include these essential nutrients in your diet and adopt a brain-friendly lifestyle; you're also nourishing your mind for a lifetime of robust cognitive health. Cheers to a joyful and healthy journey of the brain!

CHAPTER TWO

Memory-Boosting Elements

Herbs, Spices, and More

Greetings from the fascinating world of Memory-Boosting Elements! Join us on a sensory adventure with herbs, spices, and tasty allies that can improve memory and cognitive function in addition to pleasing the taste buds. We'll examine these gastronomic companions in further detail in this investigation, revealing the complex dance they do in the theater of your brain health.

1. The Golden Wonder of Turmeric:

   - **Active Friend:** Curcumin, a substance known for its anti-inflammatory and antioxidant qualities, is found within the golden hues of turmeric.

- **Memory Hangout:** Curcumin's advantages for the brain go beyond its eye-catching hue. Research suggests that it might help to improve memory and sustain cognitive function in general. Consider curcumin as your proactive ally on the path to optimal brain health, helping to combat oxidative stress and inflammation, two factors that silently undermine cognitive function.

2. Rosemary: Your Aromatic Companion

- **Aroma Sidekick:** Rosemary's strong, aromatic scent goes beyond its use as a culinary herb to become a lovely partner in your memory work.

- **Memory Jam:** According to research, breathing in the aroma of rosemary may improve memory and alertness. Think of rosemary as your vibrant friend who makes you aware of your surroundings and fills the kitchen with an aromatic symphony.

3. The Wise Man, or Sage:

-**Flavorful Pal:** Sage is a versatile character in your culinary drama that adds richness to both savory and sweet recipes. It has an earthy and somewhat peppery vibe.

- **Memory Chat:** Packed with anti-inflammatory and antioxidant properties, sage may be quietly conversing with your memory. It is the wise guy in your herb collection, quietly enhancing the health of your brain with its potential to improve cognitive performance.

4. Cinnamon: Your Sweet Cog Friend- Sweet Buddy: Cinnamon is your companion that

elevates both your savory and sweet recipes with its cozy, warm tones.

- **Memory Tango:** A chemical found in cinnamon called cinnamonaldehyde may be causing a memory tango in your brain. This tasty companion may be giving your meals a fiery twist—and possibly your cognitive health as well—though further research is needed.

5. Nutmeg: Your Nutty Friend:

Warm Associate: Nutmeg's warm, nutty essence is like a companion who deepens your cooking discussions and amplifies the flavor of your food.

- **Memory Banter:** Although further research is needed, nutmeg may be having a mildly amusing conversation with your brain that could have neuroprotective effects. Consider it your dependable companion, always ready to bring a nutty twist to your culinary explorations.

6. Dark Chocolate: The Delightful Partner:

- **Rich Collaborator:** Dark chocolate can be a valuable ally in your cognitive journey, thanks to its rich cocoa flavor.

- **Memory Harmony:** It's possible that the flavonoids in dark chocolate are enhancing memory and cognitive function in a delightful symphony. Think of dark chocolate as your decadent partner, adding a deep flavor to your culinary adventures and perhaps even boosting your mental health.

Adding Components to Your Culinary Repertoire That Improve Memory:

1. Daily Turmeric Tonic:

- Start the day off right with a warm turmeric tonic, a mixture of warm water, ginger, and a tiny bit of honey combined with the earthy flavors of turmeric. Thanks to the golden wonders of curcumin, this daily routine not only offers a tasty start but also acts as a friendly prod for potential cognitive benefits.

2. Oil Creations Infused with Herbs:

- Create infused oils using sage and rosemary to enhance your cooking endeavors. These oils introduce the aromatic personalities of sage and rosemary into your kitchen, whether they are used as a dressing base, drizzled over salads, or roasted vegetables. It's not just about taste; you can also include these sage herbal allies' possible cognitive advantages into your food.

3. Cinnamon Spice Magnificence:

- Drizzle a lot of cinnamon over your yogurt or morning coffee, or add it to savory foods like roasted sweet potatoes. In addition to offering a tasty twist, the warm, sweet undertones of cinnamon may also help create a memory dance in your mind.

4. The Nutty Touch of Nutmeg:

Grate nutmeg into your preferred recipes, such as creamy sauces and baked delicacies. Not only can nutmeg add a toasty, nutty flavor to your food, but it may also play a little game with your brain, possibly providing neuroprotective effects.

5. Escape with Dark Chocolate:

Snackle on a square of premium dark chocolate that has at least 70% cocoa content. This delicious adventure will satisfy your sweet taste while introducing you to the potential cognitive advantages of flavonoids in food.

In conclusion, these memory-enhancing components are more than just ingredients; they are gastronomic allies that give your meals a delightful twist while also perhaps weaving a thread through your cognitive health. While navigating your kitchen, picture it as a get-together with pals who not only improve the flavor of your dishes but may also be subtly promoting your mental health. A tasty and unforgettable trip through the world of spices, herbs, and delectable delicacies.

CHAPTER THREE

Mindful Living

Eating and Lifestyle Tips

When one practices mindful living, every action—including breathing, eating, and moving—becomes a conscious step toward living a harmonious and balanced existence. This path takes you through every facet of your life and encourages a profound understanding of how your choices impact your well-being. It goes beyond what's in your plate. As we go further into Eating and Lifestyle Tips that go beyond the surface, let's explore the subtleties of mindful living to nourish the body and the soul.

Eating With Consciousness: Eating is not a routine action but rather a sacred act of sustenance within the framework of mindful living. It pushes you to go from eating inanely to a level of acute awareness where every aspect of the eating experience is valued and acknowledged.

1. Savor Every Bite:

Hurried meals are a common consequence of our fast-paced lifestyles. Mindful eating encourages a diversion from this hurried approach. Instead, it encourages you to savor each bite slowly and fully, taking in the flavors and textures as they dance over your palate. This is about enjoying a sensory experience as much as filling your stomach.

2. Know when you're satisfied and hungry:

Pay attention to the signal coming from your body. A closer link with your inner guiding system is fostered by mindful eating. Eat when your hunger begs you to, and stop when your body signals that it is full. This intentional approach promotes a healthier connection with food by preventing overindulgence and mindless nibbling.

3. Sort Everything Out:

Eating is more than just a mechanical task; it's a sensual experience. Let your cuisine come to life in terms of appearance, smell, and texture. Use all of your senses when eating to fully appreciate the variety of flavors, textures, and colors that are offered to you. This heightened sensitivity transforms even a simple meal into a sensory feast.

Advice on Leading a Mindful Life:

Living consciously involves many facets of your daily existence, not just the meal. It's a whole approach that blends mindful practices with the ups and downs that come with living a normal life.

1. Express gratitude:

Adopt a grateful mindset in all of your daily endeavors. Make time each day to reflect on the positive aspects of your life. Recognizing and cherishing these moments, which might include a fulfilling meal, the warmth of the sun, or time spent with a loved one, promotes positivity and a sense of fulfillment.

2. Terminated During Dinner:

- The modern world is full of diversions, and we often overlook meals due to our busy schedules. Removing screens and outside distractions from your dining space is advised by mindful living. Make space for your attention to be solely on the company and food you are enjoying. This intentional stop transforms a routine meal into a thoughtful ritual.

3. Take Hydration Into Account:

- Maintaining hydration offers an opportunity to engage in mindfulness exercises. Make this a deliberate act rather than just mindlessly consuming the water. Drink some water and inhale deeply many times. Allow this tiny act of kindness to grow into a deliberate mindfulness moment that lasts the entire day. It is an easy-to-do but powerful exercise that energizes the body and mind.

4. Intent-Based Motion:

Being physically active is a prerequisite for leading an aware life. Engage in enjoyable activities that meet your body's requirements. By fostering a connection between the body and mind, mindful movement practices like yoga, dancing, or taking a rejuvenating stroll can support a comprehensive sense of well-being.

Maintaining Attention Away from Meals:

Being aware is an attitude to life that stresses intention and presence, rather than just following specific routines.

1. Purposeful Breathing

- Include mindful breathing techniques in your everyday regimen. Pause, take a few slow breaths, and concentrate on the present moment. This method serves as an anchor to help you de-stress and keeps you rooted in the here and now.

2. Establish Mindful Habits: Incorporate mindfulness into your daily routine. Try to be in the present moment when you travel, take a shower, or do housework. Daily tasks become opportunities to cultivate awareness, adding depth and meaning to your existence.

3. Sound Sleep:

- Prioritize sleep as the cornerstone of a contemplative existence. Create a calming bedtime routine, minimize screen time before bed, and ensure your sleeping environment promotes restful sleep. Maintaining emotional stability and cognitive function requires a regular sleep routine.

In short, living a mindful life involves taking intentional and purposeful steps that affect every aspect of your life. It's the realization that every moment offers an opportunity to be mindful and in the now. You may create a happy existence that reaches the core of who you are and extends far beyond the material world by implementing mindful eating and living habits.

Being mindful is not a destination but a continuous exploration of self-awareness and meaningful existence. I hope this path enables you to recognize the value of every second, savor the breadth of your encounters, and understand the essential connection between wise choices and a life well-lived.

CHAPTER FOUR

Brain-Healthy Recipes

Meals and Snacks

When it comes to the practice of mindful living, each and every action, breath, and bite becomes a deliberate step toward the cultivation of a harmonious and balanced existence. This trip is not only about the food that arrives on your plate; rather, it encompasses every aspect of your life and invites you to get a fundamental awareness of how the decisions you make affect your overall health and wellbeing. In order to nourish both the body and the soul, let's go on a complete examination of Eating and Lifestyle Tips that go beyond the surface and delve into the complexities of mindful living.

Mindful Consumption:

When considered in the perspective of mindful living, eating is not a routine activity but rather a holy act of providing nourishment. It encourages you to move away from consumption on autopilot and into a state of heightened awareness, in which each and every facet of the gastronomic experience is relished and acknowledged.

1. Take each and every bite:

In our hectic lives, meals are frequently a hastily prepared affair that we speed through. A deviation from this hasty attitude is encouraged by the practice of mindful eating. Instead, it encourages you to take your time and digest each bite, fully appreciating the myriad of flavors and sensations that present themselves to your palette. This technique is not only about satisfying the stomach but about reveling in a sensory experience.

2. Pay Attention to Hunger and Fullness:

- Tune in to the cues your body sends. Mindful eating fosters a deeper connection with your internal cues. Eat when hunger whispers and quit when your body expresses satiety. This attentive approach helps build a healthier connection with food, staying clear of overindulgence or mindless munching.

3. Engage Your Senses:

- Eating is not only a mechanical process; it's a sensory trip. Take a moment to properly see, smell, and feel your food. Engage your senses in the act of eating, allowing the rich tapestry of colors, scents, and textures to emerge before you. This heightened awareness converts a simple meal into a feast for the senses.

Lifestyle Tips for Mindful Living:

Mindful living transcends the dining table, spreading into every element of your everyday existence. It's a holistic approach that intertwines mindful activities with the ebb and flow of your life.

1. Practice Gratitude:

- Cultivate an attitude of thankfulness in your daily existence. Take a time each day to reflect on the wonderful parts of your life. Whether it's a nourishing meal, the warmth of the sun, or a shared time with a loved one, noting and enjoying these moments cultivates a positive mindset and a sense of contentment.

2. Disconnect During Meals:

- The modern world is replete with diversions, and meals often become a casualty of our hectic life. Mindful living urges you to walk away from devices and external influences during meals. Create a setting where you can focus exclusively on your food and the company around you. This intentional stop transforms an ordinary meal into a thoughtful ritual.

3. Hydrate Mindfully:

- Hydration, too, becomes an opportunity for mindfulness. Instead of blindly gulping down water, convert this act into a moment of awareness. Take a few deep breaths while sipping water, enabling this simple act to become a mindful stop in your day. It's a tiny yet powerful technique that restores both body and mind.

4. Mindful Movement:

- Physical activity is a vital aspect of mindful living. Engage in things that bring you delight and correspond with your body's demands. Whether it's a refreshing walk, a yoga session, or the rhythmic beat of dance, mindful movement connects your body and mind, developing a complete feeling of well-being.

Bringing Mindfulness Beyond Meals:
Mindful living extends beyond specific techniques; it's a method of experiencing life with intention and presence.

1. Mindful Breathing:
  - Integrate moments of mindful breathing into your day. Pause, take a few deliberate breaths, and bring your focus to the present moment. This exercise not only helps as a stress-reliever but also serves as an anchor, grounding you in the now.

2. Cultivate Mindful Habits:

- Infuse awareness into your regular habits. Whether it's washing dishes, taking a shower, or commuting, approach these chores with present-moment awareness. Mundane tasks convert into opportunities for awareness, bringing depth and purpose to your daily existence.

3. Quality Sleep:

- Prioritize sleep as a cornerstone of thoughtful life. Create a calming nighttime routine, minimize screen time before sleep, and ensure your sleep environment supports peaceful slumber. Quality sleep is a non-negotiable part of total well-being, contributing to cognitive performance and emotional equilibrium.

In essence, mindful living is a conscious and intentional journey that encompasses every part of your life. It's an understanding that each moment contains a chance for awareness and presence. By embracing mindful eating and lifestyle practices, you develop a harmonious existence that stretches far beyond the tangible, touching the heart of your being.

Mindful living is not a destination but a constant journey, an evolving discovery of self-awareness and deliberate life. As you traverse this path, may you find the beauty in every moment, appreciating the depth of your experiences, and understanding the profound connection between thoughtful decisions and a life well-lived.

CHAPTER FIVE

Holistic Well-being

Sleep, Social, and Beyond

In the tapestry of holistic well-being, the threads of sleep, social interactions, and beyond weave together to create a happy and lively life. This note is an examination into the interrelated domains of our existence, understanding that true well-being extends beyond physical health to cover the nuances of our sleep cycles, the depth of social bonds, and the larger range of influences that shape our everyday experiences.

Serenity in Slumber: The Dance of Sleep

Consider the night as a holy dance between you and the universe. Quality sleep is not only a period of rest; it's an essential performance that rejuvenates your body, nurtures your mind, and aligns your spirit. It's a delicate ballet where each sleep cycle plays a part in memory consolidation, emotional equilibrium, and overall cognitive performance. Embrace the peacefulness of a good night's sleep as the basis of overall well-being, allowing your body and mind to dance in rhythmic harmony.

The Social Symphony: Connections That Nourish

Social relationships shape the tune of our lives, generating a symphony of shared experiences, laughter, and support. These relationships are not just extras; they constitute the backbone of comprehensive well-being. Whether with family, friends, or community, the warmth of human interaction offers delight and fulfillment. In this social symphony, locate the cadence that resonates with your spirit. Nurture relationships that elevate, share in moments of vulnerability, and allow the harmonies of connection to resonate through the corridors of your existence.

Beyond the Horizon: Mind, Body, and Spirit

Holistic well-being extends its arms beyond the visible horizon. It encompasses the mind, body, and soul in a dance that involves more than simply the physical. Engage in activities that create a feeling of purpose, whether it's exploring your passions, pursuing personal improvement, or contributing to the greater good. The spirit grows when connected with ideals and meaning, producing a resonance that transcends the everyday. Embrace techniques that cultivate mindfulness, bringing your awareness to the present moment and allowing the spirit to breathe.

The Dance of Nutrition: Fueling the Body Temple

Consider the food you consume as a significant part of the overall dance. Nutrition is not simply about satisfying hunger; it's a rhythm that sustains the body temple. Embrace a broad and colorful array of fruits, veggies, nutritious grains, and lean proteins. Let each meal be a celebration of nourishment, supporting your physical well-being and contributing to the energy that fuels your dance through life.

Nature's Choreography: Outdoor Connection

Step outside and experience the ground beneath your feet. Nature is a choreographer, encouraging you to join its dance. The outdoors is not only a backdrop; it's an active participant in total well-being. Whether it's a stroll through a park, a hike in the mountains, or simply basking in the warmth of sunlight, nature's dance gives a break for the mind, a tonic for the body, and a salve for the spirit.

Harmony Within: Mindfulness and Inner Peace

Holistic well-being finds its heart in the quietude of mindfulness and inner calm. Amid the clamor of daily life, carve aside moments of silence. Whether via meditation, deep breathing, or introspective activities, develop a sanctuary within. It's a harmonious environment where you may reconnect with your soul, finding balance and tranquility in the midst of life's hectic rhythms.

In the magnificent tapestry of holistic well-being, each piece is a critical thread adding to the beauty of the whole. Sleep, social connections, mindful practices, diet, and the dance with nature are all interrelated, producing a symphony that resonates with the rhythm of life. Embrace this dance with an open heart, realizing that true well-being is a journey of harmony, balance, and the joyous celebration of your complex existence.

CONCLUSION

Lifelong Brain Empowerment

The pursuit of brain empowerment throughout life is the crescendo that plays through the years in the symphony of our existence. This trip is more than just a show; it's an ongoing investigation and a dance with the mind as it changes, grows, and matures throughout life. Let's consider the harmonies of knowledge, nourishment, and mindful living that lead us toward a future in which the mind remains resilient, nimble, and empowered as we wrap out this story on lifelong brain empowerment.

The Understanding of Wisdom:

Understanding is the first step toward lifetime brain empowerment. Recognizing the flexibility of the mind and its complex inner workings, as well as the influence of lifestyle decisions. It involves having a constant conversation with oneself, being genuinely curious, and being willing to learn new things. This wisdom turns into the cornerstone of a trip that gradually becomes clearer every day, creating a rich tapestry of insights that enhance the mental terrain.

Nutrition as a Guide:

The mind grows when it is nurtured, much like a garden does when it is well-maintained. By the decisions we make, from attentive exercises to brain-boosting diets, we supply the necessary elements for cognitive vigor. It's not just about feeding the body; it's also about creating an atmosphere that gives the mind the support and care it needs. In the future, nourishment will serve as our compass, pointing the way toward a mentally robust and dynamic society.

A Legacy of Mindful Living:

The practice of mindful living bears the imprint of lifetime brain empowerment. It's an acceptance that every choice you make affects the course of your mind, a dedication to being fully present in the moment, and a deliberate decision to cherish every experience. Being mindful is a long-term habit that incorporates intention into day-to-day activities rather than being a passing fad. It turns into a legacy that is passed down from one generation to the next— a gift of insight, fortitude, and mental health expertise.

Welcoming Lifelong Education:

The search of information becomes an enduring partner in the quest for brain empowerment throughout one's life. Learning becomes a lifetime endeavor, whether it is via formal education, the excitement of discovery, or the knowledge imparted by those who have gone before us. It's an admission that information is a never-ending source of growth for the mind, with every new insight serving as a brushstroke toward a more vibrant, capable mind.

A Resilient Symphony:

As we get to the end of this trip to equip our brains for life, picture a resilient symphony. Similar to an orchestra, the mind adjusts to the shifting beats of life, blending victories and setbacks in perfect harmony. It's a song about adjusting to the ups and downs of life with resilience, fortitude, and an unyielding spirit. Lifelong brain empowerment is a continuous symphony that plays on, leaving a legacy of cognitive vibrancy for future generations. It is not a destination.

The mind is the conductor of our life's symphony, the maestro in the tapestry of our existence. A tribute to the resiliency and potential that are present in every one of us is lifetime brain empowerment. We leave a lasting legacy when we pursue information relentlessly, cultivate the mind with intention, accept the wisdom of insight, and live mindfully. Cheers to a lifetime of empowerment where the mind explores, grows, and dances in the never-ending field of possibilities!